100

FOOD
RULES

FOR CHILDREN
UNDER 100 YEARS !

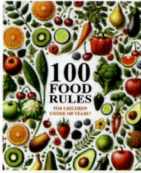

100 Food Rules

Published by Association for Human Development Inc.

First Edition: 2025

Cover design by: Srinivasa K. Rao, Ph.D.

This book is a work of non fiction.

For information about special discounts for bulk purchases, please Contact:

Srinivasa K. Rao, Ph.D.
New York, USA.
rao@food123.us

100 Food Rules | ISBN 978-1-7374931-7-4 | Price $9.99

An imprint of
Prakhya Art Printers Pvt. Ltd., India.
Ph: +91 95810 77468, print@prakhyaarts.com

Appeal

We invite you to explore and try these 100 Food Rules.

We welcome your insights and experiences in following these rules.

Feedback

Please scan the QR code
to give your feedback

Dr. Srinivasa K. Rao, Ph.D
rao@food123.us

Acknowledgment

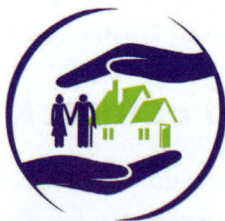

INDIA HOME
A CENTER FOR SENIOR CARE

Mrs. Geetha Jamballi
Mrs. Kavita Shah
.....and the Team

New York, USA.

Table of Contents

The Team

Ms. Lalitha Ramamoorthy, MS, RD
Ms. Anjali Singh, MA
Prabha Venkata Purnima, B.Tech.
Ms. Kanishka Upadhyay, MS
Dr. Srija Reddy, MBBS
Dr. Pramoda Prattipati, MBBS
Dr. CJK Akash Kumar, MBBS
Dr. Vaibhavi Burra, MD
Dr. Prerana Saini, MD
Dr. Tejasri Reddy, MD
Dr. Venkata Madhavi Latha Telagarapu,
MBBS, DGO, MBA, MPH.

&

Dr. Srinivasa K. Rao, Ph.D.
rao@food123.us
+1 516 859 3010
New York, USA.

Resources :

1. For Scientific Literature - https://pubmed.ncbi.nlm.nih.gov

2. International Conference on Nutrition in Medicine

3. EAT Commission

4. Encyclopedia of Herbal Medicine by Dr. Andrew Chevallier

5. 'How Not to Die' by Dr. Michael Greger

6. Food Rules by Mr. Micheal Pollan

7. Food Rules by Dr. Catharine Shanahan

100 Food Rules
for a
Healthier You

Welcome to a journey to be healthy!
With 100 rules to guide your way.

From food to fitness, mind to rest,
Each rule will help you feel your best.

Eat right on time, move with grace,
Balance in every meal you embrace.

Refresh, flex, and rest
Thrive with life, feeling best.

Tiny changes, big rewards,
Wellness is what each rule offers.

So take a breath, start today, and let
Your health lead the way!

DISCLAIMER

The information in this book is for educational purposes only and is not medical advice. It is based on general health and nutrition principles and should not replace professional medical consultation, diagnosis, or treatment. Personal health conditions should be considered before making significant dietary or lifestyle changes. Always consult your physician for the right guidance. The authors and publishers are not responsible for any adverse effects or consequences from the use of any suggestions or procedures described in this book, without the needed professional guidance.

Preface

In today's fast-paced world, the vital link between our food and our well-being is often overlooked.

We face an onslaught of conflicting dietary advice, fad diets, and ultra-processed food options.

Amid this confusion, the enduring wisdom of traditional practices and the clarity of modern science shine as guiding lights.

This book seeks to merge age-old knowledge with contemporary research, offering a comprehensive guide to eating for better health.

How to Use This Book

1. **Start Small :** Begin by integratinga few rules into your daily routine. Small, consistent changes can give good results.

2. **Personalize Your Journey :** Choose the ones that resonate with your goals, lifestyle, andpreferences.

3. **Involve Your Loved Ones :** Share these rules with family and friends to foster a collective journey towards health and happiness.

4. **Use the** "Top Foods For Better Health" tables given on pages 102-107.

1

Use Food As a Medicine

Treat food as medicine to stay healthy and prevent disease, reducing the need for medications.

2

Think Beyond Genetics

Remember healthy habits like diet, exercise, and strong social connections play a role in health in addtion to genetics.

3

Follow Personalized Nutrition

Eat a well-balanced, personalized diet as each body is unique.

4

Maintain a Healthy Weight

Keep healthy weight, because overweight increases the risk of several diseases.

5

Avoid Fad Diets

Choose a balanced, sustainable diet for long-term health over extreme or trendy fad diets.

6

Stay Engaged with Learning

Keep learning about
food and nutrition
to improve your
understanding and
to stay healthy.

7

Listen to Your Body

Adjust your diet based on how your body feels - cut down on foods that cause digestive issues and increase those that boost energy.

8

Follow Body Rhythm

Understand your body's natural rhythm that affects your overall health, so try to eat and sleep at regular times.

9

Follow a Structured Daily Routine

Wake up early, practice yoga, and eat light, fresh foods can improve physical and mental well-being.

10

Start the Day with Water

Start your day with a glass of water to support hydration, kidney function, and overall well-being.

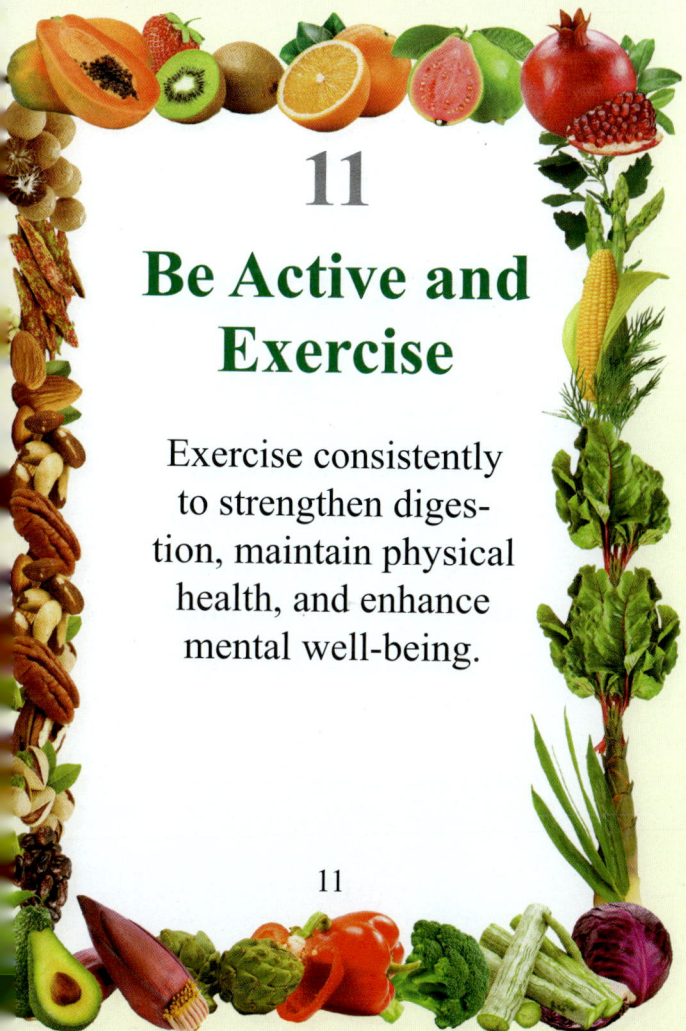

11

Be Active and Exercise

Exercise consistently to strengthen digestion, maintain physical health, and enhance mental well-being.

12

Get Enough Sunlight

Expose yourself to sunlight daily to align your biological clock and maintain adequate Vitamin D levels.

13

Manage Stress for Better Health

Learn to manage minor, sustained stress levels, using relaxation methods which can improve health.

13

14

Prioritize Sleep for Better Eating

Ensure adequate
sleep, as poor
sleep can lead to
overeating and
unhealthy
food choices.

14

15

Plan Your Meals

Plan meals ahead to ensure healthy options are readily available, reducing the temptation for fast food.

16

Balance All Six Tastes in Your Diet

Include sweet, sour, salty, bitter, pungent, and astringent tastes daily to promote balance and overall health.

16

17

Space Out Meals

Avoid frequent
snacking; evenly
spaced meals help
maintain stable energy
and blood sugar.

18

Plan Your Plate

Fill your plate half with fruits and vegetables, a quarter with protein, and a quarter with grains.

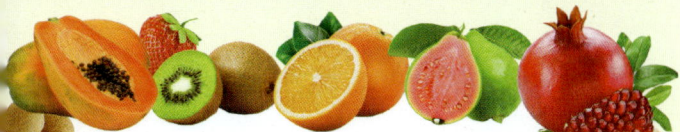

19

Count Your Calories

Consume food based on your calorie needs; multiply carbs/protein by 4 and fats by 9, then total accordingly for daily intake.

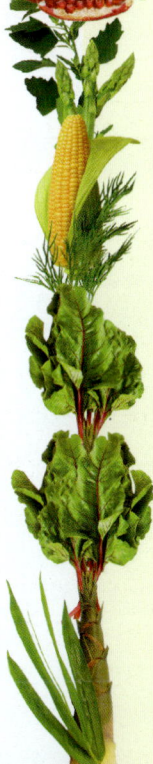

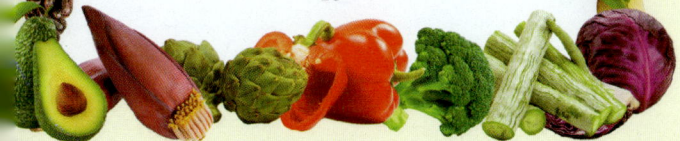

20

Balance Calories

Get 45-65% calories
from carbohydrates,
10-35% from protein,
20-35% from fats,
basedon your
calorie need.

21

Practice Portion Control

Be mindful of portion sizes, especially with high-calorie foods, to avoid overeating.

21

22

Use Smaller Plates

Use smaller plates
and bowls to
manage portion
sizes while still
feeling satisfied.

23

Practice Mindful Eating

Pay attention to flavors, textures, and hunger cues, avoiding distractions like screens, to enjoy food fully.

24

Chew Food Thoroughly

Take time to chew
food completely for
better digestion.

25

Maintain Good Posture

Sit upright while eating to aid digestion, prevent overeating, and improve overall comfort.

25

26

Move After Meals

Take a brief walk or light activity, post-meal to boost digestion and healthy blood sugar.

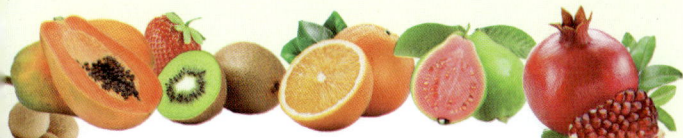

27

Don't Skip Regular Meals

Don't skip meals:
It's important to eat
regularly to keep your
body fuelled and
healthy.

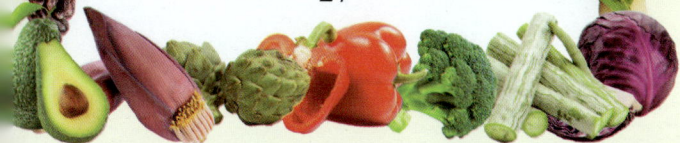

28

Avoid Late - Night Eating

Try to finish your last meal at least two to three hours before bedtime to aid digestion and sleep quality.

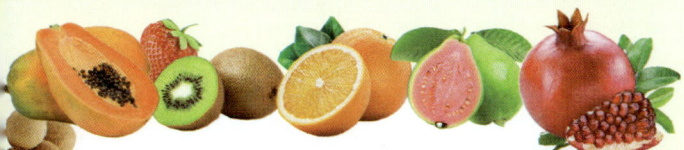

29

Fast for
Better Health

Fast for a minimum
of 18 hours in a
day to improve
metabolic health
and prevent lifestyle
diseases.

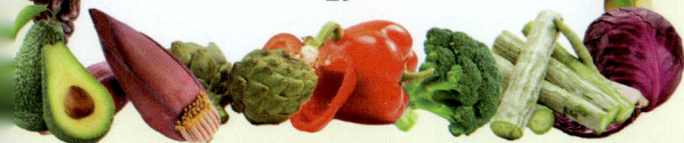

30

Favor Plant-Based Foods

Eat a more
plant - based diet
to complement
natural digestion
and supports better
health.

31

Prioritize Low Glycemic Index Foods

Choose foods with a glycemic index of 55 or lower to maintain steady blood sugar levels and sustained energy.

32

Boost Immunity

Strengthen your
immune system by
eating foods high
in vitamins and
minerals like
papaya, spinach, and
sweet potatoes.

33

Support Vision Health

Consume Vitamin A-rich foods to protect your eyesight and prevent night blindness, especially important as you age.

34

Prioritize Antioxidant-Rich Foods

Incorporate antioxidant-rich foods like berries, nuts, and leafy greens as omega-3 sources to support the brain and general health.

34

35

Consume Fiber-Rich Foods

Eat fiber-rich foods like vegetables, fruits, and whole grains to support digestion, and prevent constipation.

35

36

Distribute Fiber for Balance

Distribute fiber intake evenly throughout the day to prevent gas, bloating, and digestive discomfort.

36

37

Eat a Rainbow of Fruits and Vegetables

Incorporate fruits and vegetables of different colors for a variety of nutrients and antioxidants.

37

38

Include Fermented Foods

Consume probiotics, fiber-rich foods, and fermented foods like yogurt, kimchi, and sauerkraut to nourish beneficial bacteria and enhance digestion.

39

Eat Whole Fruits

Choose whole
fruits over fruit
juices for the added
fiber and reduced
sugar content.

40

Choose Whole Grain Snacks

Snack on whole
grain foods like
popcorn or whole
grain crackers.

41

Try Nutrient Dense Grains

A whole grain like quinoa that gives protein, fiber, vitamins, and minerals can replace rice and wheat.

42

Try Different Millets

Experiment with different types of millets, such as pearl millet, finger millet, and proso millet for added variety and nutrients.

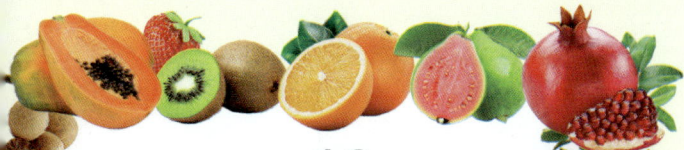

43

Soak Your Grains and Legumes

Soak grains and legumes to reduce anti-nutrients, enhance nutrient absorption, and improve digestibility.

43

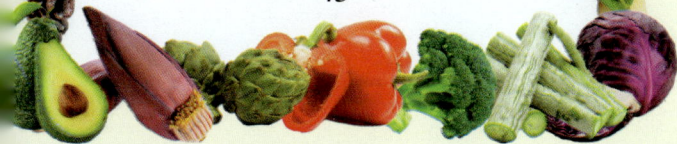

44

Use Lentil Power

Include lentil or
bean soup daily,
choosing from 40
different pulses for
protein, fiber, and
essential nutrients
to boost health.

44

45

Rotate Your Protein Sources

Include a variety of
protein sources such
as beans, legumes,
tofu to diversify
nutrients.

46

Pair Carbs with Protein

Combine high-carb
foods with protein or
fiber for steadier blood
sugar and
lasting energy.

47

Eat Seasonal Foods

Eat foods suited to the season. For example, brinjals and tomatoes are best consumed in winter, not in summer.

48

Use Produce Peels

Use all edible peels of fruits and vegetables for their nutrients and fiber after thourghly cleaning them.

48

49

Eat Hydrating Fruits and Vegetables

Select fruits and
vegetables that
contain high
water content which
contribute to your
hydration.

49

50

Choose Fresh or Frozen Foods

Choose fresh or frozen fruits and vegetables over canned foods, which can contain added sugars, salts and preservatives.

51

Include Leafy Greens Daily

Make leafy greens like spinach, kale, and arugula a regular part of your meals for essential micro nutrients.

52

Incorporate Traditional Remedies

Learn how to use simple, traditional remedies like herbal teas for common ailments like colds, coughs, and digestion problems.

52

53

Include Traditional Recipes

Utilize family and regional traditional diets that have been used for generations.

53

54

Prefer Home - Cooked Food

Home-cooked meals are healthier, fresher, and more nutritious than restaurant or fast food options.

55

Wash Before You Chop

Wash fruits and vegetables before peeling or chopping to avoid losing nutrients.

56

Try New Cooking Methods

Experiment with grilling, baking, or stir-frying to introduce new flavors and textures.

57

Cook Food Thoroughly

Cook all food items thoroughly to kill bacteria.

58

Eat Cooked Foods Promptly

Consume cooked foods within 4-6 hours; if left out, reheat thoroughly before eating.

59

Ignite Kitchen Creativity

Experiment with flavors, colors, and textures to make healthy food choices exciting and enjoyable.

60

Eat Fat to Get Thin

Healthy fats boost metabolism, curb hunger, and balance hormones, aiding fat loss when consumed mindfully with balanced meals.

61

Consume Healthy Fats

Use nuts as a
snack instead of
junk food to get
healthy fats.

62

Use Healthy Oils in Cooking

Choose healthy oils like olive oil, avocado, and nut oils and clarified butter in cooking.

63

Balance Different Oils

Use a combination
of oils like rice
bran, sesame,
groundnut, olive
to meet all your
nutritional needs.

63

64

Reduce Fried Foods

Limit the intake of
fried and fatty foods
help reduce
heart attacks, stroke
and cancer risk.

65

Avoid Reusing Cooking Oil

Avoid reusing cooking oil to prevent harmful chemicals and reduce cancer risk.

66

Eat More Berries

Eat berries,
like blueberries
strawberries or others
for their antioxidant
anti-aging and
health benefits, choosing
from 40+ berries.

67

Replace Sugary Snacks

Cut down on sugary snacks and choose natural options like fruits.

68

Avoid Sugary Drinks

Limit consumption of sugary beverages like sodas and sweetened juices.

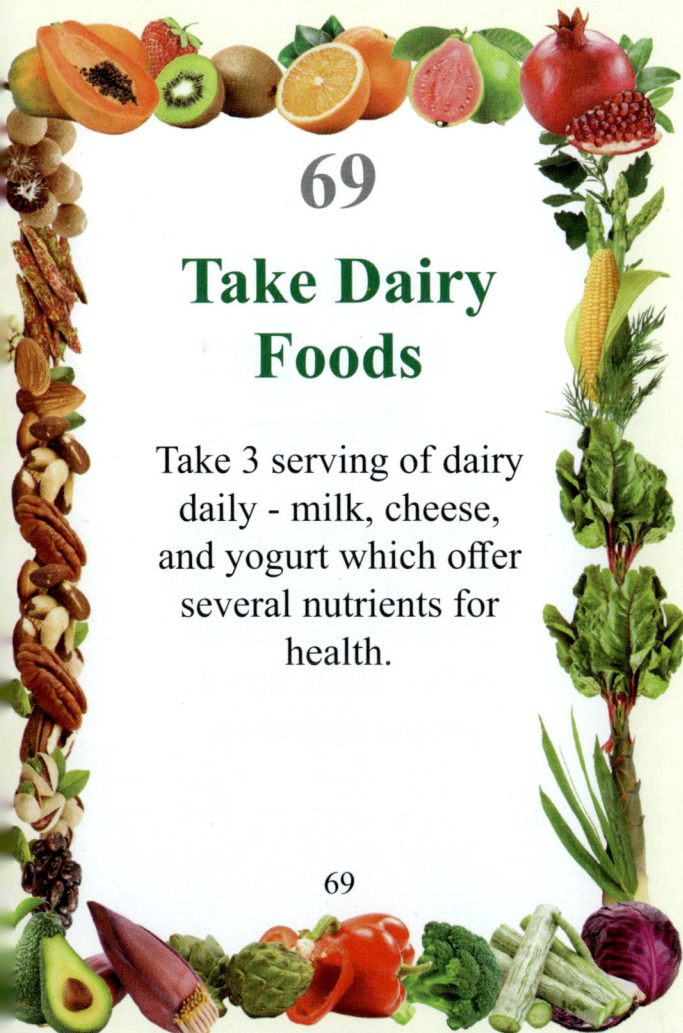

69

Take Dairy Foods

Take 3 serving of dairy daily - milk, cheese, and yogurt which offer several nutrients for health.

70

Drink Enough Water

Drink enough water
daily and check urine
color—light yellow
or hay color signals
proper hydration.

71

Drink Water When Exercising

Stay hydrated by drinking water before, during, and after physical activity.

72

Drink Coffee and Tea in Moderation

Enjoy coffee and tea in moderation, which offer some health benefits.

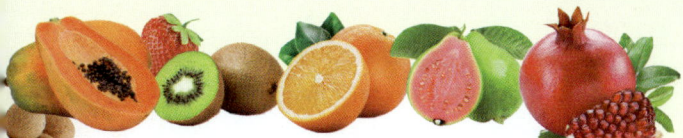

73

Drink
Herbal
Teas

Enjoy herbal teas
like chamomile or
peppermint to support
healthy digestion and
restful sleep.

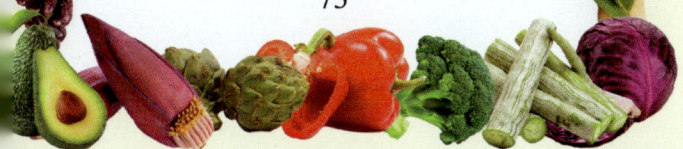

74

Drink Green Tea

Make green tea
a regular part of
your diet for its
antioxidant benefits.

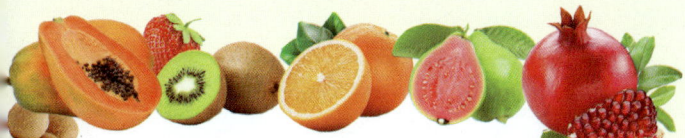

75

Avoid Tea With Meals

Avoid drinking tea along with a meal because it interferes with absorption of iron and calcium in the body.

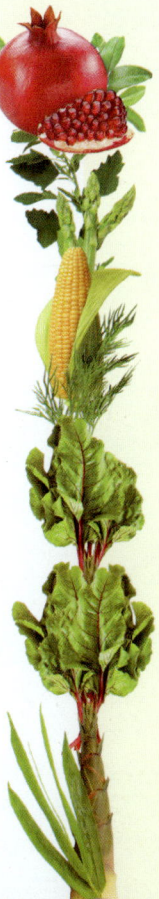

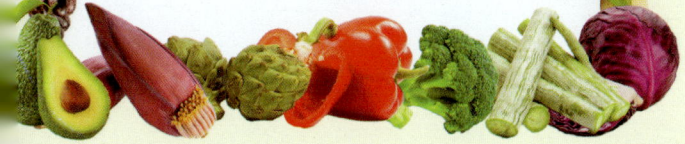

76

Crunch on Veggie Chips

Swap regular snacks with veggie chips for a healthier, and tasty way to increase your vegetable intake.

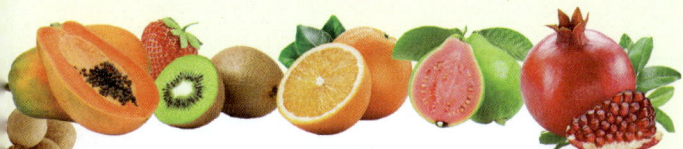

77

Use Veggie Noodles

Replace regular noodles with veggie noodles to boost vegetable intake and add nutrients to your meals.

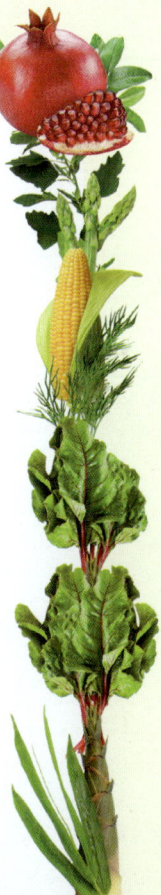

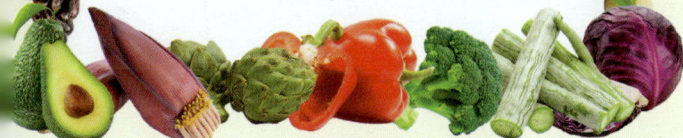

78

Eat Minimally Processed Foods

Fresh, minimally
processed foods
are more nutrient-dense
and beneficial
for health.

79

Avoid Spicy Foods

Spicy foods cause irritation to the stomach lining, increasing the risk of ulcers and stomach cancer.

80

Eat Sour Foods for Digestion

Consume sour foods like lemon and yogurt to stimulate digestion by producing saliva and breaking down food.

81

Eat Astringent Foods for Tissue Health

Astringent foods like pomegranate and berries tighten tissues, aid digestion, reduce inflammation, promote detoxification, regulate blood sugar, and provide antioxidants.

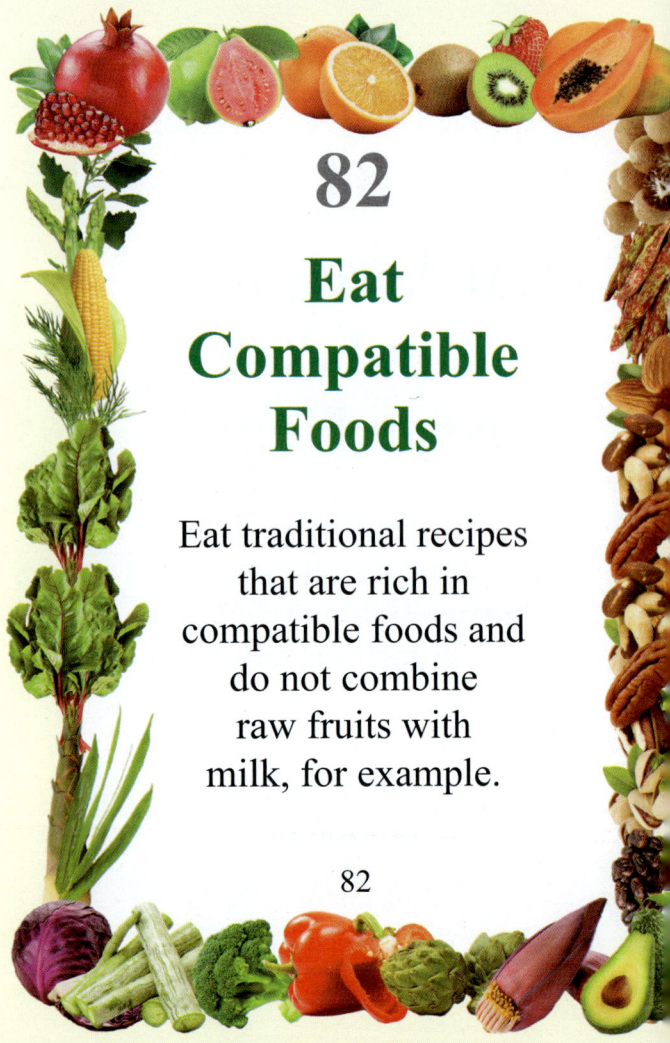

82

Eat
Compatible
Foods

Eat traditional recipes
that are rich in
compatible foods and
do not combine
raw fruits with
milk, for example.

82

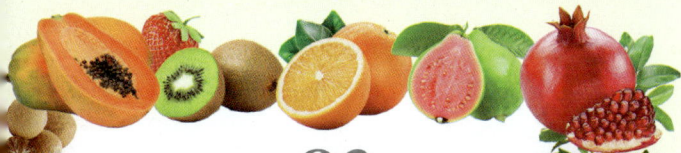
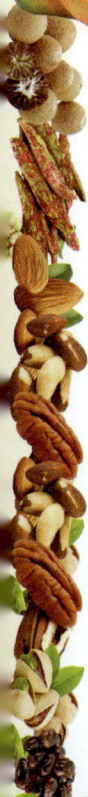
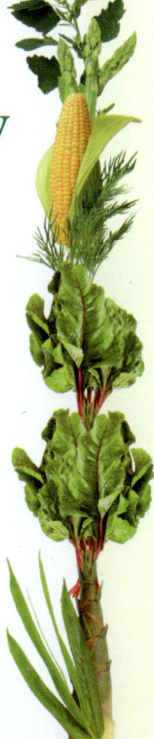

83

Stock Healthy Foods in the Kitchen

Keep your kitchen
stocked with
healthy food items.

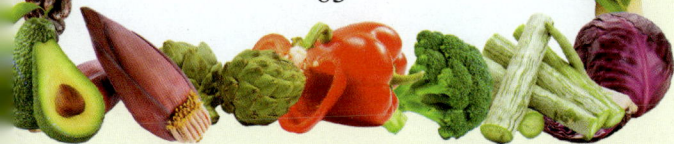

84

Store Food Properly

Refrigerate perishable foods and store as per the storage conditions appropriate for each food item.

85

Minimize Plastic Use for Health

Store and heat food in stainless steel or glass containers to reduce microplastic exposure and protect your health.

86

Read Food Labels

Read the food labels on packaged food and check the ingredients and nutritional facts and expiry date before consumption.

86

87

Check Labels for Hidden Sugars

Read food labels to check for added sugars and avoid them.

88

Opt for Fortified Foods

Choose foods fortified with essential vitamins and minerals like Vitamin D, Iron, Iodine, and Vitamin A to meet nutritional needs.

89

Check Allergen Info on Labels

Always read allergen information on food labels to avoid allergic reactions and ensure safe eating.

90

Consume Before the Expiry Date

Ensure food is consumed before the expiry or best before date to avoid health risks from expired products.

91

Limit Salt Intake

Reduce the use of
salt in cooking and
adding to foods.

92

Limit Alcohol Consumption

If you consume alcohol, do so in moderation, and opt for red wine for potential health benefits.

93

Limit Processed Meats

Reduce the intake of processed meats like sausages, bacon, and deli meats, which are linked to increased health risks.

94

Follow Variety for Vitality

Enjoy a diverse range of plant foods from over 1,000 options to maximize nutrition and health benefits.

95

Have Regular Health Checkup

Stay aware of your body's changes and· consult healthcare professionals for regular checkups and adjust your food accordingly.

95

96

Get Your Gut Microbiome Tested

Regularly test your gut microbiome to understand its health, enabling personalized dietary adjustments for optimal digestion and overall well-being

96

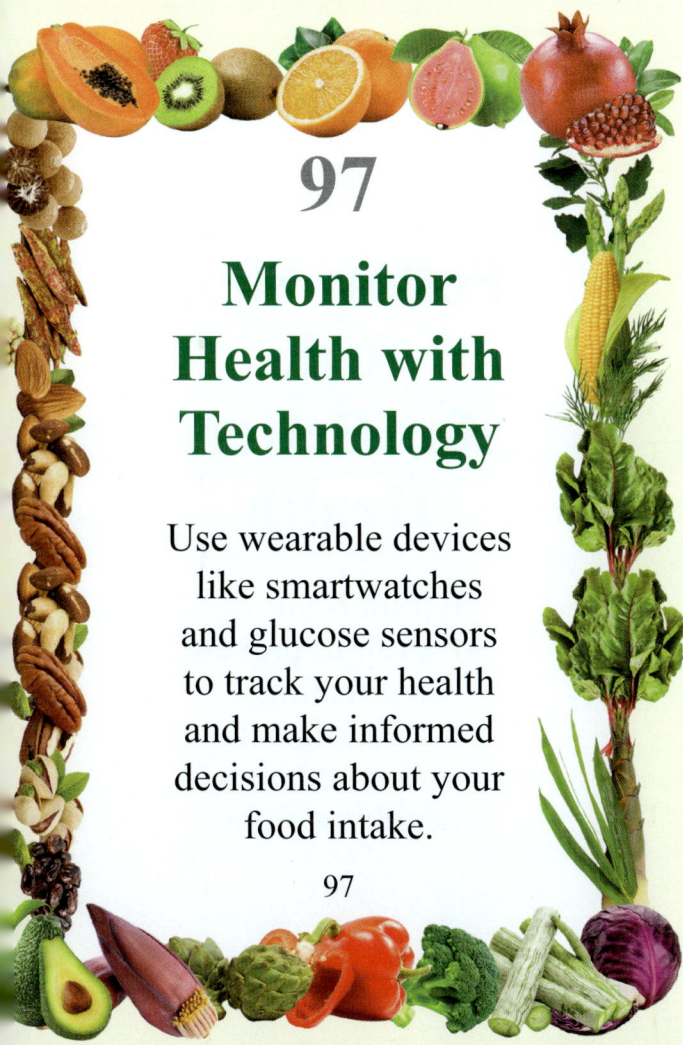

97

Monitor Health with Technology

Use wearable devices like smartwatches and glucose sensors to track your health and make informed decisions about your food intake.

97

98

Follow 80% Rule for Better Health

Eat until you're
80% full to prevent
overeating,
promote digestion,
and maintain a
healthy weight.

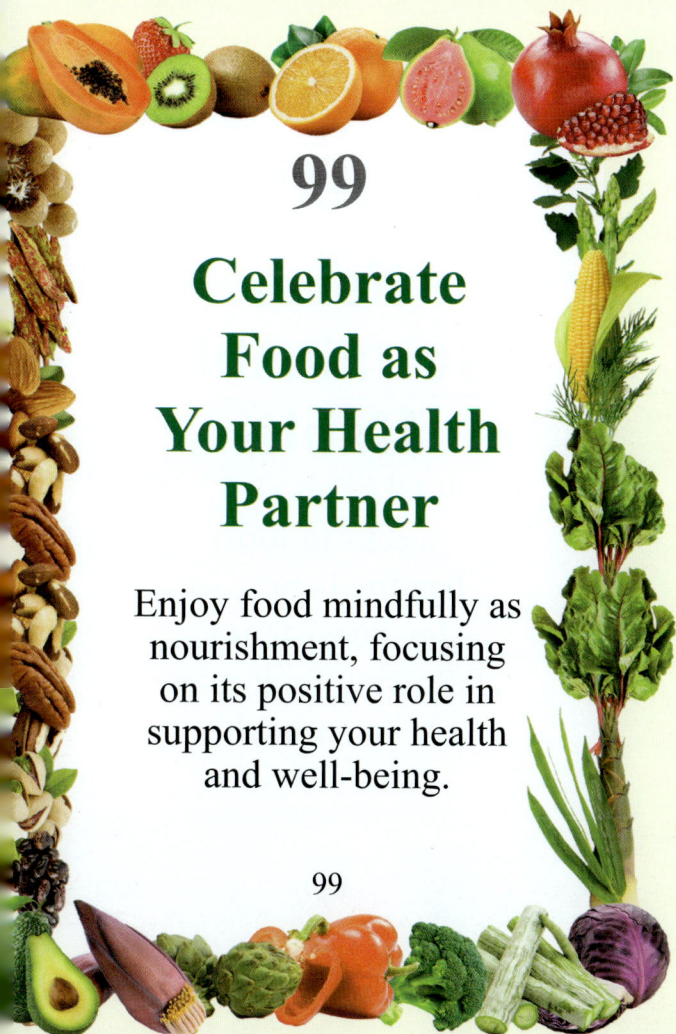

99

Celebrate Food as Your Health Partner

Enjoy food mindfully as nourishment, focusing on its positive role in supporting your health and well-being.

100

Form Sustainable Habits

It takes about 12 weeks to form healthy habits, so stay consistent in fallowing food rules for better health.

TOP
FOODS
FOR
BETTER
HEALTH

For ANTIOXIDANTS

1. Pecan
2. Walnut
3. Chia
4. Hazel nut
5. Pear
6. Cranberries
7. Cranberry beans
8. Kidney bean (dark red)
9. Pink Beans
10. Prunes
11. Coffee
12. Pinto bean
13. Black Lentils
14. Artichoke
15. Plum
16. Blackberry
17. Raspberry
18. Chestnut
19. Blueberry
20. Pomegranate
21. Almond
22. Black-eyed Beans
23. Strawberry
24. Raisins
25. Dark Chocolate
26. Fig
27. Quinoa
28. Apple
29. Red cabbage
30. Lotus root

For CALORIES

1. Macadamia
2. Pecan
3. Walnut
4. Brazil nut
5. Piyal seeds
6. Coconut
7. Hazelnut
8. Almond
9. Pinenut
10. Cashew
11. Hemp Seeds
12. Pistachio
13. Groundnut
14. Niger seeds
15. Gingelly
16. Chia
17. Safflower seeds
18. Cacao
19. Flax seeds
20. Linseeds
21. Oats
22. Common Millet
23. Buckwheat
24. Lupin Beans
25. Teff
26. Soya bean white
27. Chickpea
28. Spelt
29. Rye
30. Barnyard Millet

For FIBER

1. Chia
2. Cacao
3. Flax seeds
4. Linseeds
5. Soya bean white
6. Lupin Beans
7. Black Matpe
8. Cranberry beans
9. Pink Beans
10. Pinto bean
11. French beans
12. Yellow eye beans
13. Gingelly seeds
14. Split yellow pea
15. Green peas
16. Marrowfat peas
17. Kidney bean (dark red)
18. Brown Lentils
19. Curry leaves
20. Barley
21. Coconut
22. Mung bean
23. Rye
24. Quinoa
25. Moth bean
26. Barnyard millet
27. Almond
28. Safflower seeds
29. Dried goji berries
30. Farro

For GI (LOW)

1. Broccoli	10	16. Chickpeas	28
2. Cabbage	10	17. Lentils (boiled)	29
3. Mushrooms	10	18 Black Beans	30
4. Almonds	10	19. Greek Yogurt	33
5. Peanuts	14	20. Pears	38
6. Spinach	15	21. Green Peas	39
7. Cauliflower	15	22. Carrots	39
8. Zucchini	15	23. Apples	39
9. Asparagus	15	24. Oranges	40
10. Tomatoes	15	25. Plums	40
11. Bell Peppers	15	26. Strawberries	41
12. Walnuts	15	27. Milk	41
13. Cherries	22	28. Peaches	42
14. Kidney Beans	24	29. Sweet Potato	44
15. Grapefruit	25	30. Blueberries	53

For IRON

1. Niger seeds
2. Pearl Millet
3. Barnyard Millet
4. Gingelly seeds
5. Cacao
6. Quinoa
7. Dried acai
8. Little Millet
9. Curry leaves
10. Soya bean white
11. Piyal seeds
12. Moth bean
13. Chia
14. Amaranth
15. Teff
16. Black Matpe
17. Red lentils
18. French green lentils
19. Green Lentils
20. Raisins
21. Raisins
22. Dried goji berries
23. Mung bean
24. Chickpea
25. Garden cress
26. Cashew
27. Parsley
28. Flax seeds
29. Linseeds
30. Amaranth Leaves

For PROTEIN

1. Soya bean white
2. Lupin Beans
3. Hemp Seeds
4. Black Matpe
5. Groundnut
6. Mung bean
7. Black Lentils
8. French green lentils
9. Green Lentils
10. Red lentils
11. Pistachio
12. Gingelly seeds
13. Brown Lentils
14. Pigeon peas (Tur)
15. Split yellow pea
16. Green peas
17. Marrowfat peas
18. Kidney bean (dark red)
19. Moth bean
20. Chickpea
21. Flax seeds
22. Linseeds
23. Niger seeds
24. Piyal seeds
25. Cashew
26. Cranberry beans
27. Pink Beans
28. Pinto bean
29. French beans
30. Yellow eye beans

Mark the Completed Rules

1	11	21	31	41	51	61	71	81	91
2	12	22	32	42	52	62	72	82	92
3	13	23	33	43	53	63	73	83	93
4	14	24	34	44	54	64	74	84	94
5	15	25	35	45	55	65	75	85	95
6	16	26	36	46	56	66	76	86	96
7	17	27	27	47	57	67	77	87	97
8	18	28	38	48	58	68	78	88	98
9	19	29	39	49	59	69	79	89	99
10	20	30	40	50	60	70	80	90	100